Cannabis Extract Guide

The Ultimate Guide On How to Make Marijuana Extracts For Cooking in Your Home, Including Cannabis Cookbook With 10 Recipes for Tasting Cannabis Cookies

Monica Jacobs

©**Copyright 2016 by Monica Jacobs - All rights reserved.**

This document is geared towards providing exact and reliable information in regards to the topic and issue covered. The publication is sold with the idea that the publisher is not required to render accounting, officially permitted, or otherwise, qualified services. If advice is necessary, legal or professional, a practiced individual in the profession should be ordered.

From a Declaration of Principles which was accepted and approved equally by a Committee of the American Bar Association and a Committee of Publishers and Associations.

In no way is it legal to reproduce, duplicate, or transmit any part of this document in either electronic means or in printed format. Recording of this publication is strictly prohibited and any storage of this document is not allowed unless with written permission from the publisher. All rights reserved.

The information provided herein is stated to be truthful and consistent, in that any liability, in terms of inattention or otherwise, by any usage or abuse of any policies, processes, or directions contained within is the solitary and utter responsibility of the recipient reader. Under no circumstances will any legal responsibility or blame be held against the publisher for any reparation, damages, or monetary loss due to the information herein, either directly or indirectly.

Respective authors own all copyrights not held by the publisher.

The information herein is offered for informational purposes solely, and is universal as so. The presentation of the information is without contract or any type of guarantee assurance.

The trademarks that are used are without any consent, and the publication of the trademark is without permission or backing by the trademark owner. All trademarks and brands within this book are for clarifying purposes only and are the owned by the owners themselves, not affiliated with this document.

Table of Contents

Introduction 5

Chapter 1: A Brief Guide to Growing Cannabis 6

Chapter 2: A Brief History of Eating Cannabis 11

Chapter 3: Cannabis Extraction Methods 15

Chapter 4: Cooking with Cannabis 22

Chapter 5: Cannabis Cookie Recipes 26

Conclusion 37

Introduction

I want to thank you and congratulate you for purchasing the book, "Cannabis Extract Guide".

This book contains proven steps and strategies on how to make Cannabis Extracts and Cannabis Cookies in your home like a pro.

While some of you may already be quite happily growing cannabis in your back garden or down in the cellar, there will be those who don't know where to start. I will give you a brief guide on how to grow your own cannabis, but for the most part, this book will concentrate on cannabis extraction methods and baking the most delicious cookies with your cannabis extracts.

Thanks again for purchasing this book, I hope you enjoy it!

Chapter 1: A Brief Guide to Growing Cannabis

When it comes to growing your own cannabis, there are several steps that you need to follow for success. This is a brief guide to how to grow your own cannabis:

1. **Choose your location**

Are you growing indoors or outdoors? Indoor growing is a more private endeavor because it is away from prying eyes and it also gives you a higher level of control. It is also relatively cheap to set up an indoor cannabis farm, especially if you just want a couple of plants to keep you going. You can grow cannabis in a spare room, in your garage, in your basement, even in a closet.

One of the most important things about growing cannabis is to control your temperature although that isn't always possible if you choose to grow outside. Young cannabis plants need more warmth and will grow quicker when your temperatures are set to between 70 and 85° F – don't forget that, when your lighting is installed, that will raise the temperatures a little. When your plants are older, they will do better with cooler temperatures – between 65 and 80° F. This will help to produce the best buds.

Growing cannabis outdoors is even cheaper because the environment will do a lot of the work for you and you won't need to pay out for lighting or heating. However, you do need to keep an eye on things – if you live in a hot, dry climate, you will need to water your plants whereas, if your climate is rainy, you need to protect your plants from getting too much water.

2. Lighting

If you are growing indoors, there are several different types of lighting to choose from:

- CFL – compact fluorescent light bulbs
- LED grow lights
- Other fluorescent bulbs
- MH - Metal halide
- HPS - High-pressure sodium

Your plants need at least 8 hours of light per day so if growing outside they must be in direct sunlight for a minimum of 8 hours, preferably between 10 AM and 4 PM as this is when the sun is at its strongest and warmest.

If growing indoors, choose your lighting carefully. HPS and MH lights are the gold standard and provide the best overall lighting environment. They are powerful and cheap to buy and set up, as opposed to the LED lights, which are incredibly expensive. Many beginners start with CFL and move on to stronger lights for the flowering season

3. Growing Medium

Choose your growing medium carefully because each one has different requirements. The most common mediums are:

- Organic composted soil, full of nutrients
- soilless mixes – coco coir, vermiculite, perlite, etc.
- hydroponic – combined with MH or HPS lights, this provides the best and fastest growing medium

4. Nutrients

The type of nutrient required depends on the type of growing medium you are using. If you are using the composted soil, specifically made for cannabis plants, you will already have sufficient nutrients for the first stage of growing. From here on, and for those who are using hydroponic or soilless mediums, you will need to purchase specifically formulated cannabis nutrients. Alternatively, you can use something like Dyna-Grow at half strength. Dyna-grow is a two-system nutrient – one for the vegetative stage and one for the bloom stage.

As with all nutrient systems, don't start at full strength because you can burn your plants. You only need to raise the dose if your plants develop a problem like yellowing leaves or leaves dropping unless this occurs in the last couple of weeks before you harvest.

Always test the pH of your plants, which means testing your water before you introduce it. If you use composted super soil, you don't need to do this, as the microbial life in the soil will take care of the plants for you. Purchase a testing kit and stick to these general rules:

- For soil - 6.0 - 7.0
- For hydroponics – 5.5 – 6.5

5. The plants

If you know other growers, you can easily get your plants and know that they are a good strain. If you don't, you will need to purchase good quality seeds – you can do this online. You can also buy clone plants.

6. Seed Germination

If you have clone plants this section is irrelevant to you. For seed germination, the best way is to purchase a starter cube; keep it moist and warm and when the seedling appears you can put the entire cube into your chosen growing medium.

Another way is to place your seeds on paper towels on a plate, moisten it and cover with another plate. When the seedlings appear, you can transplant them.

7. Vegetation State

Once your plants have their first set of leaves they are classed as being in the vegetative stage. Keep the temperature constant and water regularly. Ensure that they have 18-24 hours of light per day if growing indoors and are in the strongest direct sunlight if growing outdoors.

8. Flowering

When your plants begin to bud, they are in the flowering stage. At this point, you will need to determine if your plants are male or female and discard the males. The males do not produce buds, only pollen sacs and are useless. You can ensure you get females by purchasing female clones or feminized seeds. You also need to change your lighting to 12 hours on and 12 hours off if growing indoors.

9. Harvesting

When your buds no longer produce new white hairs on them, you should be able to smell a strong cannabis smell. Wait for at least 40% of the hairs to turn a darker color and curl in – from here you can start harvesting. For the highest levels of THC (more about this later), harvest when between 50 and 70% of the hairs are dark.

10. **Drying and curing**

Hang your harvested buds' upside down in a dark and cool space with lots of ventilation so they can dry out. They should dry slowly and do make sure to check regularly for mold. Your buds are dry when the thin stems snap and the bigger stems are still a little bendy so now it's time to cure them to ensure a good smooth flavor.

Place the buds into mason jars, tightly closed and stored in a dark and cool place. Fill the jars ¾ full. Every day for the first 2 weeks, open the jars for a few seconds. This allows air in and moisture out. If your buds are moist, leave the lids off until they feel dry to the touch.

When the buds have been dry for at least 7 days, you can go down to removing the lid once a week. Cure for up to 30 days.

Chapter 2: A Brief History of Eating Cannabis

The very first drink with an onomatopoeic name was bhang because of the effect of your head feeling like it is exploding as you down it. Originating in India in the 10th century, bhang was the first product from experimentation with cannabis and its narcotic properties. By 1580, bhang was the most popular drink ever. But how was it made?

The leaves and the buds of the cannabis Sativa plant were ground using a mortar and pestle into a green paste and were then mixed with ghee, milk, and spices. Another recipe involved the boiling of the leaves first but the rest of the method was pretty much the same with the buds and leaves being mashed and mixed with sugar and water. These were then formed into small balls, names bhang goli, that were used as an aid to sleeping and consumed as an appetizer.

At around the same time, cannabis for cooking was also catching on in Europe. Bartolomeo, an Italian scholar from the 15th century published a book by the name of "On Honorable Pleasure and Health" and this contained a ganja recipe. Written in Latin, the recipe translates as:

"To make cannabis yourself more commonly used as flax for thread, use a mallet to crush clods [buds?] collected after a good harvest. Add cannabis to nard oil in an iron pot, crush together over some heat and liquefy into a health

drink of cannabis nectar. Carefully treat food and divide for the stomach and the head. Finally remember everything in excess may be harmful or criminal."

Even back then, in the 15th century, Platina was already beginning to talk like one of our modern-day potheads! And, if you can find a picture of him standing beside the Pope of the time when he was appointed to the Vatican, take a look at the eyes of both men – they look somewhat glazed!

Platina used heat as a way of rendering the THC but the Indians didn't do this so, is it possible that you can eat raw cannabis and still get high? The answer is yes, you can. It is an absolute myth that cannabis has to be cooked in oil or butter and that myth was totally debunked by a native of San Francisco, Alice B Toklas (1977 – 1967). Toklas was highly famous for her cooking and also for her cannabis baking, among friends such as Picasso, Hemingway, Matisse, and Paul Bowles. Bowles wrote, *"The user of cannabis is all too likely to see the truth where it exists and to fail to see it where it does not"*.

We can only assume that Toklas gave her friends some of her well-known hash brownies, the recipe for which appeared in her 1954 book, The Alice B Toklas Cookbook. While this won't be seen as an issue by any pot heads, the problem with the recipe, called Hashish Fudge, was that it contained absolutely no hash whatsoever and neither did it have any chocolate in it. Toklas did not come up with the recipe herself; instead, it came to her via Brion Gysin, a performance artist, painter, and a friend of William S Burroughs. Also, there is no baking in this recipe – the ingredients are simply mashed together and rolled into balls, similar to the bhang goli from India. The recipe reads:

"Take 1 teaspoon black peppercorns, 1 whole nutmeg, 4 average sticks of cinnamon, 1 teaspoon coriander. These should all be pulverized in a mortar. About a handful each of de-stoned dates, dried figs, shelled almonds, and peanuts: chop these and mix them together. A bunch of cannabis Sativa can be pulverized. This along with the spices should be dusted over the mixed fruit and nuts, kneaded together. About a cup of sugar dissolved in a big pat of butter. Rolled into a cake and cut into pieces or made into balls about the size of a walnut, it should be eaten with care. Two pieces are quite sufficient."

So yes, cannabis can be eaten raw and this recipe is of no small historic importance. Unfortunately eating raw cannabis does lead to another problem – constipation – so it isn't really advisable.

Of course, the hippies love the recipe and it made its mark in the Peter Sellers film called, *I Love You Alice B Toklas.* The movie is centered on a lawyer who eats a hash brownie or two and then disappears from his wedding, running off to live with a hippie. These were depicted as real brownies and this is why the brownie became the food of choice to infuse cannabis into and this is how it became associated with Toklas, albeit erroneously.

As with any cannabis cooking, the secret to good pot brownies is experimentation though Some people use butter, while others choose peanut oil because it has a much higher smoke point than butter. To cut costs you can use leaves that have already been used in the production of bubble hash and, once you have rendered the THC into the fat, use a brownie mix in a box and just add it into the ingredients.

Cannabis is not limited to brownies, though! You can use it in a wide range of foods and if you go to any medical cannabis dispensary you will find a range of cookies, lozenges, fig bars, lollipops, and cakes. In fact, if you use it at home, you can use it in just about cooking you want, especially if you use it in the form of canna oil or cannabutter.

There are plenty of websites that are dedicated to cooking with cannabis and plenty of books, all of which give you, not just delicious recipes to try but a whole load of medical advice with it. That said, you don't need special recipes; just chuck it in your cooking and enjoy.

A couple of years ago, Roberta's Pizzeria in Bushwick held a hush-hush cannabis feast that made it into GQ magazine. They served a full gala meal that included cocktails with a cannabis base, a salad of vegetation that was grown on their roof and bluefish that was seasoned with canna oil and served in a cannabis yogurt sauce. Two different pizzas were served, both made from hempseed dough, seasoned with 'herbs' and pot pesto. And the desserts, way too numerous to mention, included vanilla tuille made with cannabutter, a hempseed crumble and a strawberry-rhubarb gelato that was served with cannabis cream.

Of course, this does pose one question – just how high can you get?

Chapter 3: Cannabis Extraction Methods

Cooking with cannabis is fun, a wonderful way to pep up your favorite recipes. However, it isn't just a case of crumbling a bud into your ingredients; you need to do a bit of planning first and that means learning the art of cannabis extraction. Cannabis contains something called THC, or tetrahydrocannabinol and this is soluble when you place it into an oil-based solvent. The THC is what is responsible for the feel-good factor of cannabis consumption but you cannot blend this straight into your cookie recipes. It has to be extracted first but, before you can do that, it needs to go through the act of decarboxylation.

This is a crucial part of using cannabis in food. To get the true value of the cannabis, it has to be heated up to a temperature that is not achievable in our digestive systems. There is a downside to this process – some of the aromatics that are responsible for the flavor and aroma will be lost. You can try adding raw material to the decarboxylated material in equal quantities but this is a matter for experimentation.

The Decarboxylation Process

Be warned – you will have an extremely strong cannabis smell throughout this process!

Once you have cured your buds they are ready for the decarboxylation process:

1. Preheat your oven to 225° F
2. Get a rimmed baking tray or an oven-safe dish and line it with parchment paper
3. Break the buds into small pieces and place them in an even layer in the tray or dish – do not overlap any but keep them close together
4. Bake in the preheated oven for about 20 minutes – this is to remove moisture so do keep an eye on them. The plant color should turn from a light to a dark brown shade and, when ready, should look crumbly
5. Set aside to cool and turn the heat in the oven to 240° F
6. Crumble the cooled cannabis bud evenly over the base of the dish and cover it with aluminum foil. Make sure to crimp the edges to create a tight seal
7. Bake for between 45 and 60 minutes
8. Remove and leave to cool off completely before you remove the foil
9. If the finished material is very fine you can use as is; if not, blend until fine but do not over blend – you don't want a fine powder
10. Store in a glass airtight container in a dry and cool place until you need it.

Infusion Methods

There are 3 main infusion methods to get your cannabis ready for use in your cooking:

Canna Oil

Ingredients:
- 6 cups of extra virgin olive oil
- 1 oz. fine ground cannabis bud

Instructions:
1. Use a double broiler or a heavy-bottomed pan to heat the oil slowly for a few minutes – the aroma of the oil will begin to appear
2. Add a little of the bud and stir to coat it; continue adding the bud slowly until it is all mixed in
3. Simmer for about 45 minutes on a low heat, stirring on occasion
4. Remove and cool before you strain it
5. Use a fine metal strainer and press the bud against it with a spoon to get all of the oil out of it
6. Recycle the used solids on the compost heap and store the oil in the refrigerator in an airtight container for up to 2 months

Cannabutter

Ingredients:
- ½ oz. decarboxylated cannabis bud
- 1 lb. unsalted butter
- 4 cups water

Instructions:
1. Cut the butter into small pieces and combine with the water and the cannabis bud in a pan
2. Heat over a low heat – do not boil, just simmer for 3 to 4 hours
3. Stir the mixture every half hour or so – it will begin to thicken so don't let it become too thick. The cannabis should be floating around 2 inches off the base of the pan and should never, ever, touch the base. If needed, add a little more water
4. After a few hours, the mixture should be dense, more compact and look glossy. Turn the heat off and leave to cool
5. Line a metal sieve with two cheesecloth layers, allowing some overhang
6. Pour the cooled mixture into the sieve, using a spatula to press it down into the cloth. Leave to drain over a bowl
7. Wearing gloves, bring the cheesecloth corners together and squeeze the butter out by twisting it
8. Discard the cannabis residue in the cloth and use a spatula to remove any butter left in the pan into the bowl
9. Refrigerate for about 2 hours until the butter has turned solid

10. When cooled, use a knife to separate the edges of the solidified butter and lift it from the bowl. Place it wet side facing up onto a cutting board and mop off any excess water – expect your butter to have a slight green tinge to it
11. Store in an airtight container in the refrigerator until ready to use – do not keep for more than a couple of weeks

Canna Coconut Oil

Ingredients:
- ¼ to ½ oz. decarboxylated cannabis bud
- 1 cup organic coconut oil – use cold-pressed

Instructions:
1. Lay out a piece of 10 inches by 8-inch cheesecloth
2. Layer the cannabis evenly over a small area in the center of the cloth
3. Fold two opposite ends over to cover the cannabis
4. Fold one of the remaining open ends in, tuck it and roll the cloth
5. Tie the roll with cooking twine, making sure it is tight
6. Fill the bottom of a double broiler with a few inches of water and place the second pan on top
7. Turn the heat to medium – the water must reach a gentle boil, never a rolling boil
8. Put the coconut oil in the top pan. When it has melted almost completely, add in 1 cup of water, enough to cover the cannabis packet when you add it
9. Continue to heat until the oil is completely melted and then put the cannabis packet in. Press it down using the back of a spoon
10. Cover the broiler and leave cooking for about 90 minutes. Check on it every 30 minutes or so to make sure it is only boiling gently and that the water doesn't evaporate.
11. After about 90 minutes, the mixture of water and oil should be a deep green so turn the heat off and remove the cannabis packet; place it in a bowl and press it firmly with a spoon to get out any trapped oil.

12. When it has cooled off completely, you can squeeze it by hand as well
13. Add this oil to the rest and put it all in the refrigerator to cool off
14. When it has cooled, the water and the oil will separate – the oil should be a nice solid green color. Poke a couple of holes in it gently, place your hand over the top and drain the water off gently
15. Store in a glass airtight container until ready to use

Chapter 4: Cooking with Cannabis

Before you begin cooking with cannabis, you really need to understand the percentages of THC in the cannabis. On average, most cannabis strains have around 10% THC but all are different so make sure you find out what your strain percentage is. Let's say that you have 7 grams of cannabis or ¼ oz. Each gram of cannabis bud has a dry weight of 1000mg. If you have an average strain, with 10% THC, your THC weight would be 100 mg. As such, it would be safe to assume that, in terms of cooking 1 g of cannabis bud will have around 100 mg of THC in it.

Using this, you can find out how much TCH your particular strain of cannabis has per serving. Measure the ground cannabis and convert the measurement into milligrams. Divide that amount by the yield of the recipe to work out what the serving dose of THC is. Assuming you are making cookies, let's say an average recipe produces 60 cookies. You use 3 g of the cannabis which, divided by 10, is equal to 300 mg of THC. Divide that by the yield, in this case, 60, and you have 5 mg of THC per cookie.

Before you start cooking with cannabis, ensure that your kitchen area is properly prepped first. Use proper commonsense kitchen rules and be safe. Have a set of utensils and pans set aside purely or use in cooking with cannabis, to make sure there is no risk of cross-contamination and do make sure that your kitchen is well ventilated – this is an incredibly aromatic process!

A Note About Edibles

Eating cannabis with foods that are rich in fat and protein will ensure the cannabis effects last longer, whereas if you consume it in a candy or sugary form it won't last so long. Once you have consumed a cannabis edible, wait a period of 2 hours. If your high isn't there, don't be tempted to consume another edible – that will result in potential overdosing Simply eat something that is fatty to raise the cannabis effects. If you feel a bit too buzzed, drink a citric juice to bring your blood sugar up and counter the effects.

Cannabis Cooking Tips

The real secret to becoming a cannabis chef is practice. You will make mistakes and there will be disasters so before you get ready to cook for your guests, cast your eyes over these tips:

1. Remember that cannabis is fat-soluble; it is not water-soluble. For the THC to be released it has to be heated with fat, such as oil or butter.

2. Measure out the food you use in your recipes is important, just as it is in any recipe. You will more than likely have guinea pig testers so take it easy and use just ½ gram of THC per person.

3. Do not overheat your cannabis. Although heat is needed to release the THC, overheating can damage some of the cannabinoids. Cook for longer periods but at temperatures of below 330°F. Do NOT use the microwave!

4. Flavor is important so always test and be ready to improve on your recipes. Your cooking shouldn't have the single aim of creating a high; it should also taste nice too. Cannabis works a little like any normal herb – it will work with other herbs and, used in the form or oil or butter, is not overbearing.

5. Choose your moment for producing cannabis-infused cooking. Don't serve up a cannabis Christmas dinner, unless your guests are potheads! Ensure that your meal is served in a place where people can relax and enjoy what comes next

6. Do tell your guests what you will be serving them WELL AHEAD of time. Don't spring surprises on them because not everyone is receptive to using cannabis. Some people may even have adverse reactions to it or have certain food allergies or intolerances.

7. We know that, when eaten, cannabis can take an hour or two to have the desired effect. However, there will always be someone who can't wait for their high and will want more. This can be dangerous so make sure that every person is given a fair amount and never let anyone have a second portion

8. If a person reacts badly to cannabis ingestion, there are certain things you should do. Panic attacks or anxiety are best dealt with by leaving the person in a calm place, talking softly to them to tell them that the symptoms will disappear. The only other adverse effect that a person may experience is a sudden drop in blood pressure. They should be laid on the floor

with their knees raised up to above head level. If in doubt, call emergency services

9. Make sure you serve your cannabis meal in a relaxed atmosphere and have some good topics to hand for after-dinner conversation. Have the right music and soft drinks available for that inevitable thirst. Try to arrange it so that your guests stay overnight to avoid them driving under the influence.

10. Cannabis and alcohol don't mix very well so drink no more than one glass of wine with the meal – do not get drunk. Cannabis works very well with both coffee and chocolate so have these on hand for your guests.

Chapter 5: Cannabis Cookie Recipes

Marijuana Oatmeal Cookie Recipe

Ingredients:
- 8 ox canna oil or melted cannabutter
- 1 ¾ cup flour
- ¾ tsp baking powder
- ¾ tsp baking soda
- ¼ tsp nutmeg
- ½ tsp cinnamon
- ½ tsp salt
- 1 ½ cups soft brown sugar
- ¼ cup white sugar
- 2 eggs
- 2 tsp vanilla
- 1 cup chopped or whole raisins
- 3 ½ cups rolled oats

Instructions
1. Preheat your oven to 350° F
2. Whisk the flour, baking powder, baking soda cinnamon, nutmeg and salt together
3. Beat the butter or oil in a separate bowl with the sugar, vanilla, and eggs
4. Combine the dry and wet mixtures together and then add the oats and raisins. Stir until a smooth consistency is reached
5. Grease two cookie sheets and spoon out the dough in equal piles, about 3 inches apart. Press to flatten
6. Bake for about 7 to 10 minutes, until the cookies are brown
7. Remove from the oven and leave to stand for a couple of minutes before turning out onto a wire rack to cool

No-Bake Chocolate Cookies

Ingredients:
- 2 cups sugar
- ½ cup cannabutter
- ½ cup cocoa
- ½ cup milk
- 1 tsp vanilla
- ½ cup peanut butter
- 3 cups quick-cook oatmeal

Instructions:
1. Mix the cocoa, sugar, butter, and milk together in a saucepan and bring to the boil
2. Boil for one minute and then remove the pan from the heat. Stir the vanilla, peanut butter, and oatmeal in until combined
3. Drop spoonsful of the mixture onto greaseproof paper and leave to cool for at least half an hour before consuming

Cannabutter Cookies

Ingredients:
- 1 ½ cups all-purpose flour
- ½ cup white sugar
- ½ cup cornstarch
- 1 cup cannabutter

Instructions:
1. Preheat your oven to 375° F
2. Combine all the ingredients together until well mixed
3. Divide into balls of about 2 inches
4. Place the balls onto a greased cookie sheet and flatten with a fork
5. Bake until light brown, about 13 to 15 minutes and cool before serving

Cannabis Cinnamon Roll Cookies

Ingredients:
- 10 packs of cinnamon roll instant oatmeal
- 1 tsp baking soda
- 1 cup brown sugar firmly packed
- 2 cup cannabutter, softened
- 2 eggs
- 2 cups all-purpose flour
- ¼ cup water
- ¾ cup white sugar

Instructions:
1. Preheat your oven to 350° F
2. Mix both sugar with the butter until you have a creamy mixture
3. Beat the eggs in and add the baking soda and flour, mixing well to combine
4. Add the oatmeal packs and the water
5. Stir until the ingredients are evenly mixed to a cookie dough consistency
6. Make into small round balls and put onto a greased sheet
7. Bake for about 12 minutes or until golden brown
8. Transfer to a plate for cooling

Cannabis Ginger Cookies

Ingredients:
- 2 cups self-raising flour
- 2 tbsp. ground ginger powder
- ¾ tbsp. ground cinnamon
- ½ tbsp. ground cloves
- ¼ tsp salt
- ¾ cup cannabutter
- 1 cup white sugar
- 1 egg
- 1 tbsp. water
- 4 tbsp. molasses

Instructions:
1. Preheat your oven to 350° F
2. Sift the ginger, flour, baking soda, cloves, cinnamon and salt together
3. Cream the butter with the sugar in a separate bowl and beat the egg in. Add the molasses and water, and stir to mix
4. Add the dry ingredients gradually, stirring to combine
5. Spoon the mix onto plastic wrap and roll into a sausage shape
6. Leave for about 30 minutes to harden off
7. Slice the roll into rounds about 1 inch thick and place them onto an ungreased sheet, about 2 inches apart. Flatten each round a little
8. Back for about 8 to 10 minutes and then leave to cool for 5 minutes before transferring to a wire rack

Chocolate Peppermint Cannabis Crinkles

Ingredients:
- 4 oz. chopped unsweetened chocolate
- ¼ cup cannabutter
- 2 tsp instant coffee granules
- 1 ½ cups all-purpose flour
- ½ cup cocoa powder, unsweetened
- 2 tsp baking powder
- ¼ tsp salt
- 4 eggs
- 2 cups white sugar
- 1 tsp vanilla
- 12 oz. peppermint chips
- ½ cup powdered sugar

Instructions:
1. Heat a double broiler over water that is barely simmering and place the butter and chocolate into the top
2. Heat until both have melted, stirring constantly
3. Add the coffee, stir, and remove from the heat.
4. Stir the cocoa powder, flour, salt and baking powder together and set to one side
5. Mix the eggs, granulated sugar, and the vanilla together, beating to a light color
6. Fold the chocolate mix in and then add the rest of the dry ingredients (except for the powdered sugar), leaving the peppermint chips until last
7. Use plastic wrap to cover the dough and refrigerate for 2 hours or until the dough has firmed up

8. Preheat the oven to 325° F and grease two baking sheets
9. Sift the powdered sugar onto a plate or a small bowl
10. Divide the dough into balls of about ½ inch and then roll each ball in the sugar
11. Place the balls onto the sheets, 3 inches apart
12. Bake one tray for about 13 to 17 minutes or until the tops have crinkled and puffed – they cookies should feel firm to the touch. (Do not over bake)
13. Leave to cool while you bake the second sheet
14. Leave to cool for 5 minutes and transfer to a wire rack
15. For storage, place a slice of fresh bread in an airtight storage container with the cookies

Caramel Cannabis Cashew Cookies

Ingredients:

The Cookies:
- 2 tbsp. cannabutter
- 1/3 cup brown sugar, well packed
- 1 cup flour
- ¼ tsp salt

The Topping:
- ½ cup butterscotch chips
- 2 tbsp. cannabutter
- ¼ cup corn syrup
- 1 cup salted cashews

Ingredients:
1. Preheat your oven to 350° F
2. Blend 2 tbsp. of butter with the brown sugar until you have a crumb-like consistency
3. Add the salt and the flour and mix thoroughly
4. Press the mixture into an ungreased baking pan and bake for about 11 to 12 minutes
5. While the cookie mix is baking, melt the corn syrup and butterscotch with 2 tbsp. cannabutter – do not allow to boil
6. Pour the mixture over the cookie crust, add the cashews on top and leave to cool

Cannabis Peanut Butter Cookies

Ingredients:
- ½ cup cannabutter
- ½ cup peanut butter
- 1 cup sugar
- 1 ¼ cup flour
- ½ cup brown sugar
- 1 egg
- ½ tsp baking powder
- ½ tsp baking soda
- 1 tsp vanilla

Instructions:
1. Preheat your oven to 350° F
2. Melt the butter for a few seconds – it should not be hot or boiling
3. Mix with the peanut butter and then add ½ cup of flour
4. Mix well and add the brown sugar, half the white sugar, the egg, baking powder, baking soda, and vanilla; stir well to combine
5. Add the remaining flour and place the rest of the white sugar into a separate bowl
6. Shape the dough into balls and roll them in the sugar to coat
7. Place the balls onto a cookie sheet and bake for about 7 to 10 minutes, until they begin to crack on top and harden off
8. Remove from the oven and leave to cool.

Canna-Jam Cookies

Ingredients:
- 1 ½ cups flour
- 1/3 tsp baking powder
- 1/3 tsp salt
- ½ cup softened cannabutter
- ¾ cup white sugar
- 1 egg
- 1/3 tsp vanilla extract
- ½ cup powdered sugar
- 1 cup strawberry jam

Instructions:
1. Mix the flour, salt, and baking powder together and set to one side
2. Beat the butter with the sugar until fluffy and then beat the egg and vanilla in
3. Add the flour, beating to combine
4. Split the mixture into 2 and form into logs
5. Wrap the logs in plastic and leave for at least 60 minutes in the refrigerator
6. Preheat the oven to 350° F
7. Cut the dough logs into ¼ inch thick rounds and place them on cookie sheets
8. Bake until the edges are turning a golden-brown color, about 10 minutes
9. Transfer the cookies to a cooling rack and leave to cool
10. Place a tsp of jam onto a cookie and sandwich another cookie on top; repeat until all the cookies are used
11. Sprinkle with sugar before serving

Almond Canna-Cookies

Ingredients:
- 2 cups of sliced almonds
- 3 tbsp. all-purpose flour
- 1 tbsp. orange zest
- ¼ tsp salt
- ½ cup sugar
- 1/8 cup coconut oil
- ¼ cup canna coconut oil
- 2 tbsp. brown rice syrup
- 2 tbsp. full fat coconut milk
- 1 tsp vanilla
- ¼ cup of dark chocolate chips
- ¼ tsp coconut oil
- Powdered sugar

Ingredients:
1. Preheat your oven to 275° F
2. Line a couple of cookie sheets with parchment paper
3. Chop the almonds into smaller pieces and combine them with the flour, salt, sugar, and orange zest
4. Heat the oils, syrup and the coconut milk and stir until reaches a low boil; remove the pan from the heat and then add the vanilla, stirring it in
5. Add the dry ingredients gradually and then leave to cool for about 10 minutes, or until you can touch it
6. Spoon the mixture in rounds on the sheets leaving 3 or 4 inches between each one
7. Bake for about 15 to 17 minutes, turning the pan once during baking
8. Cool for 5 minutes before transferring to a cooling rack
9. Melt the chocolate chips in a double broiler and then drizzle the chocolate over the top using a fork; sprinkle powdered sugar on the cookies before cooking

Conclusion

Thank you again for purchasing this book!

I hope this book was able to help you to make your own Cannabis Extracts and Cookies and I truly hope you enjoyed the cookies, not just tasting them but making them too. Cannabis is no longer seen as the bad drug of yesteryear, at least not by everyone and it is fast becoming popular once more, as more and more places make medical cannabis legal.

Thank you and Bon Appetit,
Monica.

Made in the USA
Middletown, DE
09 April 2022